COMPLETE GUIDE TO CORNEAL TRANSPLANT

Essential Manual To Advanced Techniques, Patient Care, Recovery Tips, And Success Stories For Optimal Eye Health

DR. BRUNO HORAN

Copyright © 2023 by Dr. Bruno Horan

All rights reserved. Except for brief quotations embodied in critical reviews and certain other noncommercial uses permitted by copyright law, no part of this publication may be reproduced, distributed, or transmitted in any form or by any means, Including photocopying, recording, or other electronic or mechanical methods, without the prior written permission of the publisher.

Disclaimer:

The information provided in this book, is intended for general informational purposes only and should not be considered as professional advice.

The author has made every effort to ensure the accuracy of the information presented. However, readers are advised to consult with a qualified healthcare professional before attempting any herbal remedies or making significant changes to their wellness routine. Individual health conditions vary, and what may be suitable for one person may not be appropriate for another.

It is important to note that the author is not in any endorsement deal, partnership, or affiliation with any organization, brand, or company mentioned in this book. Any references to specific products or services are based on the author's personal experience or general knowledge and do not imply an endorsement or promotion of those products or services

Contents

CHAPTER ONE 19
  GETTING READY FOR YOUR TRIP........................19
    Choosing The Correct Physician And Clinic 19
    First Consultations And Evaluations 20
    Recognizing The Benefits And Risks...................21
    Insurance And Financial Aspects 21
    Guidelines For Pre-Operative Care 22

CHAPTER TWO 25
  CORNEAL TRANSPLANT TYPES 25
    Completely Thick (Piercing) Grafts.....................25
    Transfer Of Lamellar Tissue (DSAEK, DMEK) 26
    Synthetic Corneas, Or Keratoprostheses 27
    Deciding Which Kind Is Best For Each Patient.....28
    Improvements In Surgical Methods 29

CHAPTER THREE...31
  THE SURGICAL METHOD....................................31
    Getting Ready For Surgery................................31
    Options For Anesthesia 32
    Detailed Description Of The Procedure...............33

    Possible Issues And How To Handle Them 34

    Recovery After Surgery In A Hospital 35

CHAPTER FOUR 37

THE RECOVERY PROCEDURE..............................37

    Steps For Immediate Post-Op Care....................37

    Handling Soreness And Unease 38

    Rescheduled Visits And Progress Tracking..........39

    Getting Back To Your Regular Activities 40

    Expectations For A Long-Term Recovery 41

CHAPTER FIVE 45

CHANGES IN LIFESTYLE AND ADAPTATION 45

    Rehabilitation Of Vision.....................................45

    Adapting To Vision Changes..............................47

    Advice On How To Keep Your Eyes Safe After A Transplant 48

    Driving Limitations And Things To Think About...51

    Taking A Transplanted Cornea With You 53

CHAPTER SIX..57

PERMANENT CORNEAL TRANSPLANT CARE AND MAINTENANCE 57

    Medication Administration................................57

Frequent Check-Ups And Exams For Eyes 58

  Lifestyle Factors Impacting The Health Of The Cornea 60

  Patient Resources And Support Groups 61

CHAPTER SEVEN 63

  DANGERS AND COMMITMENTS 63

  Rejecting Cornea, The Donor 63

  The Cataracts 66

  Asymmetry And Additional Refractive Inaccuracies 67

CHAPTER EIGHT 69

  COMMON QUESTIONS AND ANSWERS 69

  Can The New Cornea Be Rejected By My Body? .. 69

  What Is The Duration Of The Transplant? 70

  Will I Still Require Contact Lenses Or Glasses? ... 71

  Can I Play Sports Or Engage In Any Other Physical Activity? 72

  How Likely Are Complications Following Surgery? 73

CONCERNING THIS BOOK

"Corneal Transplant" is a thorough and invaluable guide for anyone attempting to navigate the challenging process of corneal transplantation. The book provides readers with a basic overview of eye anatomy and the historical development of corneal transplants by methodically demystifying the intricate details of the cornea and the important reasons why a transplant might be required. It emphasizes how crucial corneal health is, laying the groundwork for readers to understand the significance of each stage of the transplant procedure.

Starting the process of a corneal transplant needs careful planning, and this book does a great job of assisting readers with the crucial pre-operative stages. It guarantees that patients are knowledgeable and ready, from choosing the best doctors and clinics to comprehending the dangers, rewards, and financial ramifications. Detailed pre-operative care instructions can help in lowering expectations and becoming ready, both physically and psychologically, for the procedure that is coming up.

The thorough examination of the many kinds of corneal transplants in the book—including full-thickness, lamellar, and artificial corneas—offers priceless insights into the possibilities. It equips readers with information that can greatly impact their treatment outcomes by clarifying the advances in surgical procedures and the standards for choosing the best kind for each patient.

A comprehensive and engrossing part of the surgical process provides a step-by-step explanation, including the preparation, anesthetic alternatives, the actual surgery, and possible consequences. By outlining clear expectations for patients and their families, this clarity demystifies the procedure and reduces anxiety. The emphasis on post-operative care and rehabilitation that follows is equally important; it provides helpful guidance on how to manage pain, get back to your regular activities, and comprehend your chances of long-term recovery.

The book addresses the unavoidable dangers and problems of corneal transplants, including glaucoma, donor cornea rejection, infection, and refractive defects. This section explains how these difficulties are usually treated, which reassures in addition to educating.

Another important topic addressed is lifestyle modifications following a transplant, including advice on safeguarding the eyes, rehabilitating eyesight, and negotiating travel and driving limitations. This useful guidance guarantees that patients may successfully maintain the health of their corneas and adjust to their new eyesight.

The success of a corneal transplant depends heavily on long-term care and maintenance, and the book offers comprehensive instructions on drug administration, routine eye exams, and identifying potential issues. The information and resources on support groups are included, which emphasizes how crucial community and continuous support are to the healing process.

To further empower patients and their families, the book provides succinct and straightforward solutions to commonly asked issues and concerns. It covers every angle to make sure readers are ready for every step of their corneal transplant journey, from the length of the transplant to sports participation and the possibility of complications.

A Comprehensive Global Transplantation

The Cornea: What Is It?

The transparent, dome-shaped layer covering the front of the eye is called the cornea. It is a window that regulates and directs light entering the eye, which is important for vision. The cornea, which is the outermost layer of the eye, contributes significantly to the optical power of the eye and serves as a barrier against dust, germs, and other hazardous substances. Additionally, it serves as a filter, blocking off some of the UV (ultraviolet) wavelengths that are most harmful from the sun.

What Could Make a Corneal Transplant Needed?

When corneal illness or injury results in impaired vision, a corneal transplant may be required. A corneal transplant may be required for several reasons, such as:

Keratoconus: This condition causes vision distortion when the cornea gradually thins and enlarges into the shape of a cone.

Fuchs' Dystrophy: A genetic disorder characterized by the degradation of the cornea's endothelium, which leads to fluid accumulation and visual impairment.

Corneal Scarring: Trauma, infections, or illnesses can leave a scar on the cornea that obstructs vision.

Infections: Severe infections can harm the cornea, including those brought on by the herpes simplex virus.

Degenerative Conditions: The clarity and function of the cornea may be affected by age-related changes or other degenerative conditions.

Complications from Prior Surgery: The cornea may be damaged by complications from prior eye surgery, requiring a corneal transplant.

Fundamental Anatomy of the Eye

Comprehending the fundamental structure of the eye aids in appreciating the importance of the cornea. The eye is made up of various essential parts:

The cornea is the transparent front window of the eye where light is focused.

Pupil: The orifice located at the middle of the iris, which regulates the quantity of light that reaches the eye.

The colorful portion of the eye that controls pupil size is called the iris.

Lens: It is located behind the iris and helps to focus light even further on the retina.

The layer at the back of the eye called the retina is light-sensitive and transforms light into electrical messages.

The optic nerve is responsible for sending visual data from the retina to the brain.

Clear vision is made possible by the cornea and lens working together to concentrate incoming light on the retina. This procedure may be hampered by corneal damage, which could result in serious visual issues.

An Overview of Corneal Transplantation's History

The practice of corneal transplantation, also known as keratoplasty, has a long history that began in the early 1900s. Eduard Zirm, an Austrian ophthalmologist, carried out the first successful human corneal transplant in 1905.

The groundwork for current corneal transplantation methods was laid by this groundbreaking procedure.

The success rates and results of corneal transplants have significantly increased over time due to developments in surgical techniques, anesthetics, and immunosuppressive medications.

Precision and success rates were greatly increased in the middle of the 20th century with the introduction of improved surgical instruments and techniques, such as the use of microscopes during surgery.

The field advanced even further with the establishment of donor eye banks in the latter half of the century, which guaranteed a more steady and constant supply of donor corneas. Modern methods like Descemet's Membrane Endothelial Keratoplasty (DMEK) and Stripping Endothelial Keratoplasty (DSEK) enable the selective transplantation of particular corneal layers, resulting in faster recovery times and better results.

The Value of Good Corneal Health

For general eye health and clear vision, corneal health must be maintained. Because the cornea is exposed to the elements, it can sustain wounds, infections, and illnesses.

Corneal injury can be avoided with proper eye care, which includes using protective eyewear, limiting UV exposure, and maintaining good hygiene.

Frequent ocular examinations can facilitate the early detection of corneal disorders and guarantee prompt treatment.

Maintaining the health of the cornea promotes the general function and well-being of the eye in addition to safeguarding eyesight.

Knowing about corneal transplantation's availability and procedure can offer hope and a route to vision restoration in situations where the corneal injury occurs.

CHAPTER ONE

GETTING READY FOR YOUR TRIP

Choosing The Correct Physician And Clinic

Selecting the appropriate physician and facility for your corneal transplant is an essential initial step. Consult an eye expert or your health care physician for advice first. Seek out a corneal expert with a great track record and many satisfied patients. Examine their credentials, their procedure success rates, and the practice's facilities. If at all feasible, stop by the clinic to see the atmosphere and the professionalism of the staff.

Take into account the clinic's reputation as well. Modern facilities with a committed staff of experts are common features of top-rated clinics. Websites for clinics, patient forums, and websites that provide medical reviews can all provide helpful information. Personal recommendations from loved ones who have had comparable operations performed might be very helpful.

First Consultations And Evaluations

The first consultation is the next step after selecting a physician. To assess if you are a good candidate for a corneal transplant, the doctor will do a comprehensive eye exam at this session. During this evaluation, your visual acuity will be measured, your eye health will be checked, and comprehensive scans of your cornea will be taken.

Bring your medical history, a list of the drugs you take now, and any records of past eye exams to your consultation. Your overall health and any underlying issues that may impact the surgery will be better understood by the doctor with the use of this information. Take advantage of this chance to ask inquiries concerning the process, recuperation, and anticipated results.

Recognizing The Benefits And Risks

Making an informed decision requires knowledge of the advantages and disadvantages of a corneal transplant. Typically, the advantages include better vision, pain alleviation, and an overall higher standard of living. Corneal transplants carry some hazards, nevertheless, like any surgical procedure: infection, corneal rejection, and anesthesia-related problems.

Talk with your doctor about these risks in greater detail. They can offer you a realistic viewpoint by supplying data and firsthand accounts. You can better assess your alternatives and get emotionally and psychologically ready for the procedure by being aware of the hazards as well as the possible positive results.

Insurance And Financial Aspects

Making a budget is a crucial step in getting ready for a corneal transplant. To find out what parts of the procedure are covered, start by getting in touch with your insurance company. While some insurance plans might only pay for a fraction of the surgery, you would still be liable for any out-of-pocket expenses for follow-up visits, consultations, or drugs.

Talk to your clinic about your choices for payment if your insurance does not cover the entire amount. Numerous clinics can put you in touch with medical loan providers or offer financing options. Budgeting for indirect expenses like time away from work, travel, and post-operative care supplies is also beneficial.

Guidelines For Pre-Operative Care

Following the guidelines for pre-operative care is essential to the success of your corneal transplant. Certain instructions based on your medical history and current state of health will be given by your physician. It is usually necessary to remove contact lenses a few weeks before surgery because they can change the curvature of your cornea.

It can be suggested that you stay away from some medications as they raise your risk of bleeding. Maintaining hydrated and eating a balanced diet might help you recuperate more quickly overall.

You won't be able to drive right after the procedure, so make plans for someone to drive you to and from the clinic the day before the surgery.

Get your house ready for your recuperation.

Store as many prescription drugs, eye drops, and other necessities as you may need in the postoperative days. Establishing a cozy and peaceful space can facilitate a speedy recuperation.

CHAPTER TWO

CORNEAL TRANSPLANT TYPES

Completely Thick (Piercing) Grafts

Penetrating keratoplasty, another name for full-thickness corneal transplants, is a procedure in which a healthy donor cornea is used to replace the damaged cornea in its entirety. Patients with extensive corneal damage from diseases like keratoconus, corneal scarring, or corneal degeneration are usually advised to have this treatment. The injured cornea is carefully removed by the surgeon throughout the procedure, and the donor cornea is sutured in its place.

The ability of full-thickness transplants to successfully treat a variety of corneal diseases is one of their benefits. But compared to previous transplants, this one has a longer recovery period and carries a larger risk of problems including graft rejection because the entire cornea is replaced.

Transfer Of Lamellar Tissue (DSAEK, DMEK)

In a lamellar corneal transplant, the healthy layers of the cornea are preserved and only the damaged layers are replaced with healthy donor tissue. Descemet's stripping automated endothelial keratoplasty (DSAEK) and Descemet's membrane endothelial keratoplasty (DMEK) are the two primary forms of lamellar transplants. Patients with corneal disorders like Fuchs' dystrophy or endothelial dysfunction, which predominantly affect the inner layers of the cornea, are frequently better candidates for these operations.

During DSAEK, the cornea's damaged endothelial layer is removed by the surgeon and is replaced with a thin layer of donor tissue that has endothelial cells that are in good health. By merely transplanting the

Descemet's membrane and endothelium, DMEK goes one step farther than DSAEK and may result in a quicker visual recovery and a decreased chance of rejection.

Synthetic Corneas, Or Keratoprostheses

Keratoprostheses, or artificial corneas, are synthetic implants used to restore corneal tissue that has been destroyed. When conventional donor corneas are unavailable or unsuitable for transplantation, these devices are usually utilized. Keratoprostheses come in a variety of forms and can be composed of biocompatible materials like silicone or polymethylmethacrylate (PMMA).

Patients who have undergone several unsuccessful corneal transplants or who have medical issues that make them unsuitable candidates for standard corneal transplantation are frequently advised to get keratoprostheses. Artificial corneas may not offer the same degree of visual quality as natural donor corneas, and while they might improve eyesight, they also come with concerns like infection and device displacement.

Deciding Which Kind Is Best For Each Patient

The level of corneal damage, the patient's general health and lifestyle, and the underlying corneal ailment all play a role in determining the best kind of corneal transplant for each patient. The ophthalmologist will evaluate these characteristics and go over the potential treatment choices with the patient during the preoperative evaluation.

Full-thickness transplantation might be the best choice for patients with problems that mostly affect the outer layers of the cornea, such as abnormalities or corneal scarring. However, patients who suffer from inner layer problems or endothelial dysfunction can benefit more from a lamellar transplant like DSAEK or DMEK.

An artificial cornea may be explored in situations where conventional corneal transplantation is not practical or successful, as in individuals with severe ocular surface disease or prior graft failures. Patients should be properly informed about the consequences of this approach, and the decision to implant an artificial cornea involves careful assessment of the potential risks and advantages.

Improvements In Surgical Methods

In recent years, there has been a notable improvement in corneal transplantation outcomes due to advancements in surgical procedures. The development of minimally invasive procedures like Descemet's membrane endothelial keratoplasty (DMEK), which enables more precise transplantation of the inner layers of the cornea and has been demonstrated to produce lower rejection rates and faster visual recovery than traditional techniques, is one noteworthy advancement.

Furthermore, better tissue processing and storage methods have produced donor corneas of greater quality and decreased graft failure rates. Pre-loaded donor tissue insertion devices are one technique that has expedited surgery and reduced the possibility of tissue injury during transplantation.

Furthermore, there is hope for future developments in corneal transplantation due to continuing research into tissue engineering and regenerative medicine. Researchers are looking at ways to use stem cells or bioengineered scaffolds to generate corneal tissue in the lab.

This might potentially lower the danger of rejection and eliminate the need for donor tissue. These developments offer patients with corneal diseases intriguing new opportunities for improving corneal transplantation outcomes and restoring vision.

CHAPTER THREE

THE SURGICAL METHOD

Getting Ready For Surgery

A corneal transplant requires careful planning to guarantee a successful and trouble-free outcome. Your ophthalmologist will first do a thorough eye exam to assess the condition of your cornea and determine whether a transplant is required.

Your eyes' general health will also be evaluated, and any possible dangers or consequences will be noted throughout this examination.

Should it be determined that a corneal transplant is the most appropriate course of treatment, you will receive comprehensive instructions on how to get ready for the procedure.

This can entail giving up specific drugs that might affect the surgery, such as blood thinners, and abstaining from food and liquids for a predetermined amount of time before the operation.

In addition, since you won't be able to drive right after the treatment, you'll need to make plans for transportation to and from the medical center. Having someone beside you to help and support you during the healing process is also crucial.

Options For Anesthesia

You will be given an anesthetic during a corneal transplant to make sure you are comfortable and pain-free the entire time. The choice you make regarding anesthesia will be influenced by several variables, such as your general health, the intricacy of the procedure, and your individual preferences.

A typical procedure is a local anesthesia, which involves injecting numbing medicine around the eyes to prevent pain perception. You won't feel uncomfortable during the procedure because the local anesthetic keeps you awake. General anesthesia is an additional choice that entails being asleep throughout the process. Your anesthetic provider will assist you choose the best course of action by going over the advantages and disadvantages of each option.

Detailed Description Of The Procedure

Typically, a corneal transplant involves a set of procedures meant to remove the diseased or damaged cornea and replace it with a donor cornea that is in good health. Here's a detailed explanation of the process:

Preparation: After your eye is cleaned and made ready for surgery, you will be placed comfortably on the operating table.

Incision: To reach the underlying tissue, the surgeon will make a precise incision in the cornea.

Removal of Damaged Cornea: The surgeon will use specialized tools to gently remove the diseased or damaged cornea, making sure to preserve as much healthy tissue as possible.

Preparing the Donor Cornea:

In the meantime, the donor cornea—which comes from a deceased person—is meticulously examined, measured, and ready for transplantation.

Transplantation: Using small stitches or an adhesive, the donor cornea is inserted into the recipient's eye and held in place.

Closure: After the donor cornea is inserted, the incisions are stitched up with temporary sutures to promote healing.

Possible Issues And How To Handle Them

As with any surgical operation, problems can occur even though corneal transplant surgery is generally safe and effective. Infection, corneal rejection, elevated intraocular pressure, and inflammation are a few possible outcomes.

Your surgeon will take several measures during the procedure and provide you with instructions for post-operative care to reduce the chance of complications. In the days and weeks that follow the treatment, you will also be closely watched to identify any early signs of complications.

If difficulties do arise, they are frequently adequately treated with prescription treatments such as antibiotics or anti-inflammatory drugs, as well as additional surgery if required.

You must show up for all follow-up sessions with your ophthalmologist to guarantee that any concerns are immediately resolved.

Recovery After Surgery In A Hospital

Following corneal transplant surgery, you will be brought to a recovery area and closely watched in case there are any early difficulties. At first, you could feel a little uncomfortable or have some blurred vision, but these should go away eventually.

After the procedure, you'll probably need to spend a brief time in the hospital to obtain post-operative instructions and treatment.

This can entail protecting the eye with an eye patch or shield, as well as utilizing prescribed eye drops to stop infection and encourage healing.

Your medical team will provide you with comprehensive instructions on how to take care of your eye at home during your hospital stay. These instructions will cover things like when to take off the eye patch, how to apply eye drops, and any activities or heavy object lifting restrictions. Additionally, they will arrange for follow-up sessions to assess your recovery and guarantee the transplant's success.

CHAPTER FOUR

THE RECOVERY PROCEDURE

Steps For Immediate Post-Op Care

It's critical to carefully adhere to post-operative care guidelines following corneal transplant surgery to promote appropriate healing and reduce the chance of problems.

Your eye will usually be covered with a covering to prevent unintentional bumps and rubbing. Wearing this shield for the first several days after the operation is advised by your surgeon. During this period, you must not touch or wipe your eye to protect the just transplanted cornea.

To prevent infection and lessen inflammation, your surgeon can recommend antibiotic and anti-inflammatory eye drops. Throughout the early recovery phase, it's critical to deliver these drops precisely as instructed, usually on a rigid schedule.

You could also be told to use lubricating eye drops to maintain a pleasant and moisturized eye.

You can have some soreness, tears, light sensitivity, or blurred vision in the early postoperative phase. These are natural symptoms that should go away as your eye heals. On the other hand, get in touch with your surgeon right away if you encounter any worrisome symptoms, including intense pain or abrupt changes in your vision.

Handling Soreness And Unease

Each person's experience with pain and suffering after corneal transplant surgery is unique. During the early phases of recuperation, pain medication may be prescribed by your surgeon to help ease any discomfort. It's critical to take these drugs exactly as directed and to abstain from exertion and activities that could make you more uncomfortable.

Using cold compresses on the closed eyes in addition to medicine can help ease discomfort and minimize swelling. To prevent irritating the surgery site, use an ice pack wrapped in a cloth or a clean, soft cloth. Additionally beneficial for reducing edema and accelerating recovery is sleeping with your head up.

Please don't hesitate to get in touch with your surgeon for more advice if you have severe or ongoing pain that doesn't go away with medicine or home cures. They can evaluate your symptoms and suggest further actions to assist you in effectively managing your discomfort.

Rescheduled Visits And Progress Tracking

It's crucial to schedule follow-up visits with your surgeon to track the development of your corneal transplant recuperation. Your surgeon will check your eye, evaluate the healing process, and modify your treatment plan as needed throughout these visits.

Follow-up appointments may be planned often throughout the early phases of recovery to monitor appropriate healing and swiftly address any issues. These consultations may become less regular as your condition stabilizes and your sight heals.

You must show up for any follow-up appointments on time and let your doctor know if anything changes or concerns you have about your eyesight or general eye health. During these visits, your surgeon may run a battery of tests to assess how well your new cornea is working and to detect any early warning signs of problems.

Getting Back To Your Regular Activities

You can progressively return to your regular daily activities as instructed by your surgeon, even though it's important to take it easy and avoid vigorous activity in the immediate post-operative time. But it's imperative to stay away from things like swimming, rubbing your eyes, and playing contact sports that could cause harm or illness to your eyes.

Until your surgeon gives the all-clear to resume some activities that involve heavy lifting or straining, you might need to take a few days off from work or restrict your workload. To get the most out of your corneal transplant, you must abide by the activity limitations that your physician prescribes.

You can experience improvements in your overall comfort and vision while your eye heals. Before exerting too much pressure on your eye, you must, however, exercise patience and give it enough time to heal.

Expectations For A Long-Term Recovery

It is important to realize that complete recovery from corneal transplant surgery might take several months to a year or longer, even though the first healing phase is crucial. Your eyesight may continue to steadily get better over this period as your eye gets used to the new cornea.

Maintaining regular follow-up meetings with your surgeon is crucial for tracking your recovery and addressing any potential problems. To improve your eyesight and general eye health, your surgeon might suggest additional procedures or therapies.

For the best eyesight after a corneal transplant, you might occasionally need to wear prescription eyeglasses or contact lenses. In close consultation with you, your surgeon will decide on the best course of action for correction based on your unique needs and preferences.

After a corneal transplant, many people see notable improvements in their quality of life and vision with the right follow-up and care.

However, it's important to have a realistic outlook on the healing process and recognize that it can take some time to see the desired results.

You may get the most out of your corneal transplant and continue to have clearer vision for years to come by adhering to your surgeon's instructions and taking an active role in maintaining the health of your eyes.

CHAPTER FIVE

CHANGES IN LIFESTYLE AND ADAPTATION

Rehabilitation Of Vision

Vision rehabilitation is a vital part of your recuperation process following a corneal transplant. It entails a set of actions meant to optimize your visual capabilities and adjust to any changes in your eyesight following surgery. Generally, your ophthalmologist will offer advice on vision rehabilitation that is customized to meet your requirements.

After the transplant procedure, your vision may initially be distorted or hazy. As your eyes become used to the new cornea, this is typical. Exercises and other activities aimed at strengthening your eye muscles and enhancing visual acuity may be part of vision rehabilitation. These drills could include monitoring moving things, focusing on objects at various distances, and honing eye coordination skills.

Vision rehabilitation may also include the use of visual aids like glasses or contact lenses in addition to physical exercises. With the use of these tools, you can improve your vision clarity and correct any residual refractive defects. After evaluating your vision requirements, your ophthalmologist will recommend the best corrective lenses for you.

Additionally, measures for managing any ongoing visual problems, including glare sensitivity or halos surrounding lights, may be included in vision rehabilitation. If necessary, your healthcare staff can offer advice on how to minimize these symptoms with specialist eyeglasses and lifestyle modifications. You can maximize your visual function and recover confidence in your ability to manage the environment around you by actively engaging in vision rehabilitation.

Adapting To Vision Changes

After a corneal transplant, adjusting to changes in vision can be a slow process that calls for endurance and patience. Your eyesight may fluctuate at first while your eyes heal and adjust to the new cornea. It's critical to allow yourself time to adjust and to share any worries or challenges with your medical team.

After corneal transplant surgery, adjusting to variations in visual sharpness and clarity is a frequent adjustment. Your vision may get better, allowing you to see objects and details more clearly, but there's a chance that residual distortion or blurriness will remain, especially in the early stages of recovery. Any worry or irritation can be reduced by realizing that these changes are typical and necessary aspects of the healing process.

Regaining depth perception and spatial awareness is another part of adapting to vision alterations. After the transplant, your vision might get better, but it might take some time for your brain to adjust and recognize visual cues correctly. Over time, these abilities can be improved by engaging in activities that call for depth perception, such as measuring distances or pouring liquids.

Changing your surroundings and daily routines may also be necessary to adapt to eyesight changes. This may be making sure your home has enough lighting, positioning furniture to avoid barriers, and utilizing contrasting colors to improve visibility. You can facilitate your rehabilitation process by making your surroundings more aesthetically pleasing by taking proactive measures to address these concerns.

Advice On How To Keep Your Eyes Safe After A Transplant

Following a corneal transplant, it's critical to take precautions to preserve your eyes and encourage healing. Specific post-transplant care instructions will be given by your ophthalmologist, but in the meantime, bear the following basic advice in mind:

Observe Your Medication Schedule: Take all oral and ocular drops as directed by your doctor. These drugs aid in the appropriate healing of the corneal transplant by reducing inflammation and infection.

Avoid Rubbing Your Eyes: Avoid touching or rubbing your eyes as this might impede the healing process and raise the risk of infection. Use the recommended eye drops to relieve itching and irritation, or gently rinse your eyes with a sterile saline solution.

Avoid Eye Injury: When participating in activities that put your eyes in danger of injury, put on safety glasses or goggles. Activities involving dust or debris exposure, such as yard work and sports, fall under this category.

Prevent Irritant Exposure: Steer clear of dust, smoke, and other allergens that may aggravate ocular discomfort or impede the healing process. If you're in an area that is smoke- or dust-filled, think about using a face mask or wraparound glasses for protection.

Maintain Good Hygiene: To lower the chance of bringing bacteria or other contaminants into your eyes, wash your hands and face. Avoid rubbing your eyes with unwashed hands and wash your hands with soap and water regularly.

Attend Follow-Up sessions: Keep track of your progress and discuss any concerns with your ophthalmologist by showing up for all planned follow-up sessions. These consultations are essential to the outcome of your corneal transplant and to identify any potential problems early on.

You can protect the results of your corneal transplant and encourage the best possible healing and visual recovery by heeding this advice and maintaining close attention to your eye health.

Driving Limitations And Things To Think About

Driving may be temporarily restricted after a corneal transplant while your vision heals and stabilizes. For your safety as well as the protection of other drivers on the road, you must abide by these regulations. Depending on your unique situation, your ophthalmologist will advise you on when it's safe to start driving again.

Your vision may be distorted or fuzzy during the first phase of recovery, which can make it challenging to see properly and respond swiftly to hazards and traffic signals. Driving when your vision is impaired puts you and other people at risk, so put safety first and don't get behind the wheel until your doctor gives the all-clear.

Your ophthalmologist may evaluate your visual acuity and peripheral vision once your vision has stabilized and improved enough to tell you if you are fit to drive safely. Taking visual field tests and having your road sign reading and object recognition skills evaluated at different distances may be part of this evaluation process.

Even after you've been given the all-clear to start driving again, it's critical to keep an eye out for any changes in your eyesight that can compromise your ability to drive safely. Get frequent eye exams to keep an eye on the condition of your eyes and to quickly address any problems. Furthermore, be aware of elements like weariness, drugs, and surroundings that can affect your eyesight.

While driving, stop at a safe spot if you notice any new symptoms or changes in your eyesight, such as glare sensitivity or trouble judging distances.

Then, don't drive again until you can do so safely. Making your driving safety and eye health a priority is crucial to avoiding collisions and guaranteeing a successful corneal transplant recovery.

Taking A Transplanted Cornea With You

It takes great preparation and thought to travel with a transplanted cornea to protect your eyes during the trip. Here are some pointers to ensure a seamless travel experience, regardless of the reason for your trip:

Pack Essentials: Make sure you include all prescription drugs, eye drops, and protective eyewear while traveling with a cornea transplant. To make sure you have these things with you for the duration of your trip, pack them in your carry-on luggage with easy access.

Protect Your Eyes: When traveling, you run the risk of exposing your eyes to dust, allergies, and dry air. To protect your eyes from UV radiation and lessen discomfort from airborne particles, put on protective eyewear or sunglasses.

Drink plenty of water. Dry eyes can be made worse by flying and changing weather, and they can hurt even more after a corneal transplant.

Drink lots of water to stay hydrated, and think about using lubricating eye drops to keep your eyes pleasant and moisturized.

Take Regular rests: To avoid eye strain and weariness, take frequent rests when starting a lengthy travel, such as a car trip or flight. This is the time to practice eye exercises, lubricate your eyes with drops, and blink often.

Plan for Medical Care: If you require assistance or medical attention while traveling, familiarize yourself with the medical facilities and eye care professionals in your destination.

In the event of an emergency, always have your emergency contacts list and pertinent medical information on hand.

Be Aware of Your Activities: When traveling, stay away from activities that can endanger the health and security of your eyes, like playing high-risk sports or swimming in chlorine pools. Select leisure activities that reduce the chance of illness or harm to your eyes.

You can travel with your transplanted cornea in safety and comfort by following these safety measures and making advance plans. Throughout your trip, put your eye health and well-being first. If you have any questions or concerns, don't be afraid to get medical help.

CHAPTER SIX

PERMANENT CORNEAL TRANSPLANT CARE AND MAINTENANCE

Medication Administration

The proper administration of post-operative medications is essential to the success of corneal transplantation. Usually, patients are administered a course of eye drops that include corticosteroids to reduce inflammation and antibiotics to prevent infection. These drugs need to be carefully taken as prescribed by the ophthalmologist. Complications like infection or graft rejection may result from noncompliance.

Additionally, patients should be informed of the possible negative effects of these drugs, including elevated intraocular pressure from long-term steroid use. It is crucial to maintain regular contact with the healthcare practitioner to swiftly handle any bad reactions and modify dosages. To make sure no doses are missed, it's helpful to stick to a medicine plan, maybe with the use of alarms or a notebook.

Frequent Check-Ups And Exams For Eyes

It is essential to have scheduled eye checkups following a corneal transplant. During these visits, the ophthalmologist can check on the healing process, identify early rejection symptoms, and evaluate the general health of the eyes. Tests including corneal topography, slit-lamp examination, and visual acuity will be conducted at these examinations to assess the integrity of the graft and the surrounding eye structures.

These examinations may be conducted often at first—weekly or monthly, perhaps—but they will progressively become less frequent as the eye stabilizes. Annual check-ups are still necessary, though, even years after the transplant, to detect issues that develop later. Rather than waiting for their next appointment, patients should always notify their doctor of any new symptoms right once.

Signs to Look Out for in Possible Problems

After a corneal transplant, outcomes can be considerably improved by being aware of the warning signals of probable problems. Any symptoms that include pain, redness, sensitivity to light, or sudden loss of vision should be treated with an ophthalmologist as away. These could be signs of infection, graft rejection, or other serious problems that need to be treated right once.

Warning symptoms can also include minor changes like fluctuating vision, new floaters, or a persistent feeling of something in the eye. By being aware of these signs and taking prompt action, small problems can be avoided before they worsen and the transplant's integrity and functionality are maintained.

Lifestyle Factors Impacting The Health Of The Cornea

Numerous lifestyle factors can impact a corneal transplant's long-term success. Patients should refrain from engaging in activities that raise their risk of eye injury, like contact sports unless they are well protected by eyewear.

It is strongly advised that smokers give up because smoking can worsen eye disorders and slow the healing process.

Ocular health is also influenced by general health and diet. Overall eye health is supported by eating a balanced diet high in omega-3 fatty acids, vitamins A, C, and E.

It's also critical to maintain proper hydration and control over systemic diseases like diabetes and hypertension.

Wearing sunglasses to defend against UV rays and limiting exposure to dust and pollution are two ways to regulate environmental concerns.

Following these dietary changes contributes to the preservation of the corneal graft's health as well as the general health of the eyes.

Patient Resources And Support Groups

Although adjusting to life following a corneal transplant can be difficult, individuals can get assistance from several organizations and support groups.

Be it online or in person, joining a support group can offer a feeling of community, practical guidance, and emotional support.

It can be immensely comforting and empowering for patients to be able to share their triumphs, coping mechanisms, and experiences in these groups.

Information about managing life after a transplant is available through educational resources offered by organizations like the Cornea Research Foundation and the American Academy of Ophthalmology.

Patients seeking information on medical, lifestyle, and psychological aspects of their recovery can consult brochures, websites, webinars, and hotlines.

By using these tools, patients can stay informed and supported, which improves their capacity to take good care of their corneal transplant.

CHAPTER SEVEN

DANGERS AND COMMITMENTS

Even though corneal transplantation is a very successful treatment, there are still risks and potential complications involved.

Comprehending these can aid patients in better preparing for the procedure and handling their recuperation.

Rejecting Cornea, The Donor

Rejection of the donor cornea is one of the biggest dangers connected with corneal transplantation. This happens when the recipient's immune system launches an attack on the donor cornea because it perceives it as alien.

Redness, sensitivity to light, blurred vision, and discomfort are some signs of rejection. Although rejection can happen at any point following the transplant, it usually happens within the first year.

Patients are usually prescribed immunosuppressive drugs, such as corticosteroid eye drops, which help to inhibit the immune response, to reduce this risk. Frequent follow-up appointments are essential for the early identification and treatment of any rejection symptoms.

Virus Infection

Another possible issue that can develop after a corneal transplant is infection. Infection is especially common during the early stages of healing in the eye.

Increased redness, discomfort, discharge, and a rapid loss of eyesight are typical indicators of infection. Strict adherence to post-operative care recommendations is crucial to reduce danger.

This entails using the antibiotic eye drops that have been given, practicing good hygiene, and abstaining from activities that could contaminate the eyes.

If an infection is detected, it is imperative to get medical attention right once because infections left untreated can have serious side effects, such as vision loss.

glaucoma

Increased intraocular pressure in the eye, or glaucoma, is a potential side effect after corneal transplant surgery. Loss of vision may result from optic nerve injury brought on by elevated intraocular pressure.

If the drainage angles of the eye are changed after surgery, or if the eye generates too much fluid during the healing process, glaucoma may result. It is imperative to regularly evaluate the pressure inside the eyes.

Medication, laser therapy, or other surgical operations may be used as treatments to bring the pressure under control and shield the optic nerve.

The Cataracts

Another potential issue following a corneal transplant is cataract formation. A cataract is a clouding of the natural lens of the eye that causes vision impairment. Corticosteroids, which are frequently recommended to stop the donor cornea from being rejected, can hasten the development of cataracts.

Cataract surgery might be necessary if the cataract progresses and causes a substantial loss of vision. This is taking out the clouded lens and putting in an artificial intraocular lens in its place.

Even after a corneal transplant, cataract surgery can typically be carried out safely; nevertheless, it does necessitate meticulous preparation and collaboration between the surgeon and the ophthalmologist.

Asymmetry And Additional Refractive Inaccuracies

After corneal transplant surgery, astigmatism and other refractive abnormalities are frequently experienced.

These happen when the newly formed cornea is not precisely round, leading to distorted or blurry vision. Both the healing process and the suturing methods used to attach the donor cornea might cause astigmatism.

Many tools, including glasses, contact lenses, or extra surgical techniques like laser eye surgery, can be used to treat refractive problems. To get the greatest visual results, scleral lenses or other specialty contact lenses are sometimes employed. To choose the best corrective technique, routine eye exams and discussions with an eye care specialist are required.

CHAPTER EIGHT

COMMON QUESTIONS AND ANSWERS

Can The New Cornea Be Rejected By My Body?

Rejection is one of the most frequent worries regarding corneal implants. The chance of rejection has been greatly decreased by medical science developments, even if your body can still perceive the replacement cornea as foreign tissue. About 10–20% of instances may result in rejection; however, this percentage fluctuates based on the patient's general health, the state of the eye before surgery, and the patient's compliance with post-operative care guidelines.

Immunosuppressive eye drops are given to patients to reduce the possibility of rejection by preventing the body's immune system from attacking the transplanted tissue. You must adhere to your ophthalmologist's recommended treatment regimen.

Pain, redness, sensitivity to light, and blurred vision are some indicators of rejection. Get in touch with your eye care professional right away if you encounter any of these symptoms. If rejection is identified quickly, early action can frequently reverse it.

What Is The Duration Of The Transplant?

A corneal transplant may require several years to heal, and in rare circumstances, a lifetime procedure. Several variables affect how long the transplant lasts, such as the patient's age, lifestyle, and level of adherence to post-operative care guidelines. Research indicates that more than 90% of corneal transplants are effective for a minimum of ten years, and many patients experience exceptional eyesight for considerably longer.

It is crucial to schedule routine follow-up visits with your ophthalmologist to assess the condition of the transplanted cornea and deal with any potential problems. Maintaining good eye health, which includes shielding your eyes from harm and preventing infections, is also essential to the transplant's durability. When engaging in activities that could endanger their eyes, patients are urged to keep their hands off their eyes and to wear protective eyewear.

Will I Still Require Contact Lenses Or Glasses?

Even while many corneal transplant patients see a noticeable improvement in their vision, most still require glasses or contact lenses for the best possible vision correction. Your original cornea may not match the shape of the transplanted cornea exactly, which could result in refractive defects including astigmatism, nearsightedness, or farsightedness.

During follow-up appointments, your ophthalmologist will evaluate your vision and may suggest corrective lenses to get the best possible visual acuity. To further enhance eyesight, other treatments like laser eye surgery may be necessary in certain circumstances. It is crucial to have reasonable expectations and realize that even while the transplant might significantly improve your vision, you can still require corrective glasses in some situations.

Can I Play Sports Or Engage In Any Other Physical Activity?

After a corneal transplant, you can usually resume sports and physical activity, but you must take particular safety measures to preserve your eyes. Particular recommendations will be given by your ophthalmologist depending on your particular situation and the kinds of activities you want to partake in.

You can usually resume non-contact sports like yoga, jogging, and swimming once your eye has healed enough—this can take a few weeks to months. When swimming, wear safety goggles at all times to protect your eyes from water and prevent infections. Wearing protective eyewear is essential for contact sports like basketball, soccer, and martial arts to safeguard the transplanted cornea from harm.

It could take longer to be able to play high-impact sports safely. Consult your physician about your intentions to receive tailored guidance on when and how to safely resume your favorite hobbies. You may safeguard your vision while remaining active by according to your doctor's advice.

How Likely Are Complications Following Surgery?

Even though corneal transplant surgery has a high success rate, problems might occur as with other surgical operations. Infection, elevated intraocular pressure, graft rejection, and issues with the stitches used to hold the replacement cornea are among the common consequences.

A dangerous but uncommon consequence that can happen if bacteria get inside the eye during or after surgery is infection. Infection symptoms include discomfort, redness, and drainage. Antibiotic treatment must be started right away to stop major eye damage.

Some people may develop glaucoma, or increased intraocular pressure, following surgery. Frequent eye exams can aid in the early detection and treatment of this illness. As was previously discussed, graft rejection happens when the body's immune system targets the cornea that was transplanted. You can reduce this risk by taking your medication as prescribed and making frequent follow-up appointments.

Last but not least, problems with the sutures that hold the cornea in place might occur. These include broken or loose stitches, which may need to be fixed with additional treatments. Effectively treating and preventing problems requires keeping lines of communication open with your ophthalmologist and following post-operative care instructions to the letter.

www.ingramcontent.com/pod-product-compliance
Lightning Source LLC
Chambersburg PA
CBHW072017230526
45479CB00008B/247